WINNIN

MW01596507

TRANSFORM YOUR BODY NOW WITH THE ISABODY CHALLENGE

DR. KEN SIMPSON
2009 ISABODY CHALLENGE GRAND PRIZE WINNER

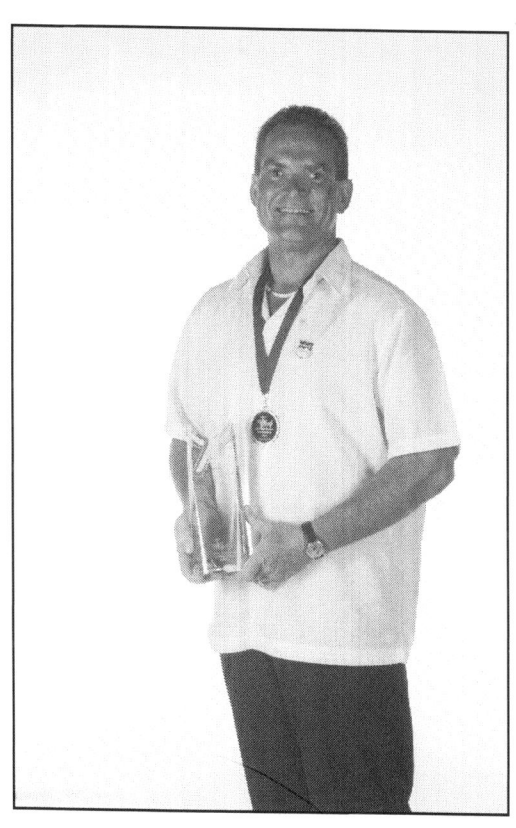

Copyright 2012 Kenneth R. Simpson, DC

ISBN: 978-1-936539-96-3

Red Willow Publishing
www.RedWillowPublishing.com

Dedications

Mindy, Lucas, Chandler, and Mekenna:
For understanding that change is 3-dimensional and
for being my reason.

Dr. Ted Brooks:
My Sponsor, My Mentor, My Friend
And for believing I could.

Rick Despain:
For his genuine love of helping people and dedication
to the continued success of the IsaBody Challenge.

The Coovers:
A lot of people have vision—very few act on it.
Fewer still ignite the same vision in others.
Your dedication to your vision allowed me to change
my life and I will remain forever grateful.

To my friends, family, patients, and Isagenix family:
Thank you for always having a word of
encouragement and love.

For the Spirit God gave us does not make us timid,
but gives us power, love, and self-discipline.
2 Timothy 1:7 NIV

CONTENTS

Introduction

I have the rare distinction of being one of only a very few people who can claim the title of Grand Prize Winner of the IsaBody Challenge. This is the body transformation competition that began in 2007 and is promoted and supported by Isagenix International LLC, the world leader in whole-body nutritional cleansing, cellular replenishing, and youthful aging. The funny thing about hearing that title is that in the beginning, I had every excuse in the book to not even start. I'll mention those excuses later on, but you need to understand that wearing the title of Winner is not where the winning began. Earning the title was an exciting point in my life's journey and I enjoyed having it bestowed on me by my peers in Isagenix, but I became a winner when I finally decided to begin the journey in the first place. That was by far the hardest part and I have respect for anyone who can finally come to the place where they make the decision to change. *That is when we truly become winners – when we finally act upon our decision to change.* Isagenix has created thousands of winners.

Chapter 1
EXCUSES, EXCUSES, EXCUSES

My friend and Isagenix sponsor, Dr. Ted Brooks, can tell you that if there was ever an excuse for not trying this program, I tried it on him. Excusitis is what I like to call it. Excusitis was my chronic cerebral inflammation of expressing my reason to avoid the change I so desperately needed. He knew of my struggles with weight for the over 10 years that I've known him and he wasn't willing to ever give up on me. I love that about Dr. Ted.

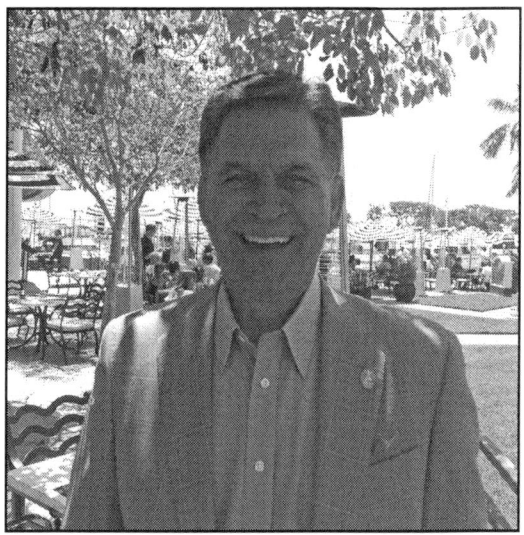

Dr. Ted Brooks

"It's too much. It's too hard. It's too inconvenient. It's not the right time in my life! I'm a doctor; what will my patients think? I already know all about nutrition. What makes you think I can't do this on my own if I want? I've tried every diet out there and then some. Why would this be any different? I've been overweight since the 4th grade; it's too late for me."

The list of excuses I threw at Dr. Ted went on and on until finally one day I said *yes* just to satisfy his desire to help and get him to stop calling me. I personally think that learning to deal with my excuses is what eventually refined the training Dr. Ted needed to become the Isagenix millionaire he is today. Anyway, that was in August of 2008 and from then through December of that year I never even tried the products. I felt like I had won because the phone calls stopped.

This is what *that* kind of winning looked like:

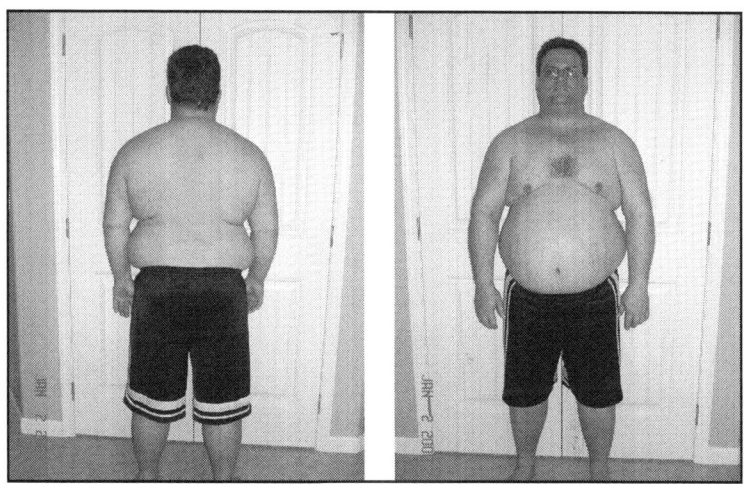

At 295 pounds I was heavier than I had ever been. I had to come up for air when I bent down to tie my shoes. I got winded walking up the stairs to tuck the kids in at night. I couldn't talk to my overweight patients about nutrition and weight loss without considering myself a hypocrite. Let's face it, I was miserable and I needed help. I had let excuses get in the way of the one thing I so desperately needed — change.

In December 2008, Dr. Ted called to tell me that Isagenix was gearing up for their 3rd IsaBody Challenge, the body transformation competition that would result in cash and prizes for the winner. *"Red carpet treatment, thousands of dollars in cash and prizes, and recognition,"* he told me. *"Oh wait,"* he said. *"I forgot you're not even using the products."* (How did he know?) *"You're probably too busy or have some other excuse,"* he said. *"I just thought you would like to know. Bye."*

How dare he think that I would have an excuse! Can you believe the nerve of some people? I was going to do this and prove him wrong. No more excuses!

When I entered the IsaBody Challenge in 2009, the format was the same as in its inception year of 2007. Its purpose was to showcase the unbelievable body transformations Isagenix had been seeing in its product users over the previous five years. In the current, upgraded version of the Challenge, participants not only get to decide on their starting date, but are eligible to earn even more cash and prizes than ever before. Now, participants can receive free products by simply remaining active in their participation for 90 days. By seeing the IsaBody Challenge through to its completion and submitting all pictures and documentation, participants are automatically enrolled in a drawing for an incredible cruise sponsored by Isagenix and the IsaBody Challenge. You can and should check all of this out and more at IsaBodyChallenge.com.

Chapter 2
ALL IN

When you make a commitment to yourself, you have to make it completely. For me, I had to stop the excuses and focus on what was necessary to succeed. I had to establish my starting point with as much documentation and information that could be tracked as possible and then create a plan. I've always heard that "if you're failing to plan, you're planning to fail." For me, failure wasn't an option. The IsaBody Challenge required photos of the beginning and end of my journey and an essay describing the transformation that included weight and inches lost, but that wasn't enough for me. I needed more if I was going to make this work every day. What did I have at my disposal that didn't cost anything and could be duplicated? How could I make sure that I was all in?

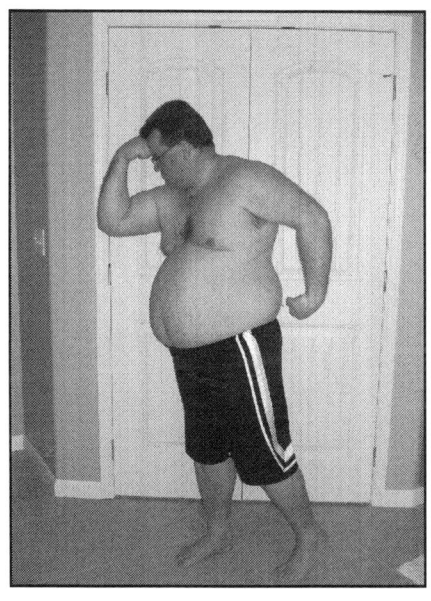

As a doctor of chiropractic, I did have some tools at my disposal that others might not have, such as a blood pressure cuff and a body fat/BMI monitor. Because I knew my history and tendencies, it was important for me to track my daily results and activities as well as my weekly and monthly progress. Since I didn't want to repeat my past failures, I made spreadsheets and charts for everything that I viewed as good health indicators. What was my blood pressure and pulse rate? What was my body fat percentage and body mass index? What was my weight and total body inches? The great thing about the different systems available through Isagenix that promote weight loss is that they also come with charts that help track your progress. I took advantage of those charts and added my own that would allow me to document the following:

What and how many calories I ate.

What times during the day did I use the Isagenix products.

How long and how much resistance training and cardiovascular exercise I did on any given day.

How my blood pressure and pulse rate were changing.

The changes in my body fat percentage and BMI.

I wanted every reason to be able to look back at any given point and see how much every single day mattered. *Every single day, I needed to make a conscious decision to succeed.*

Here is an example of additional documentation I created while at the same time using all the charts already provided by Isagenix. You can also keep track of your progress on your smartphone with the right app, tracking everything from calories to exercise to goal setting.

Dr. Ken 2009		- Weight -		295.1	& % Bodyfat -		35.8 %
Date	Day	Total Wt.	+/- Lbs.	Total Wt. Loss	% Body Fat	BMI	Fat Mass
01/02	F	295.1		N/A	35.8	43.6	105.50
01/09	F	283.1	12	12	35.1	41.8	99.5
01/16	F	275.9	7.2	19.2	34.5	40.7	95.5
01/23	F	270.1	5.8	25	34	39.9	92
01/30	F	266	4.1	29.1	33.5	39.3	89.5
02/06	F	262.9	3.1	32.2	32.6	38.8	86.5
02/13	F	255.1	7.8	40	32.9	37.7	84
02/20	F	253.4	1.7	41.7	32.9	37.4	83.5
02/27	F	246.5	6.9	48.6	31.5	36.4	77.5
03/06	F	243.2	3.3	51.9	30.9	35.9	75
03/13	F	239.7	3.5	55.4	30.5	35.4	73
03/20	F	234.3	5.4	60.8	30.2	34.6	71
03/27	F	Cruise	+1.1	C	C	C	C
04/03	F	235.1	13.4	60	30.2	34.7	71
04/10	F	230.2	4.9	64.9	29.1	34	67
04/17	F	226	4.2	69.1	27.7	33.4	62.5
04/24	F	221.3	4.7	73.8	28.4	32.7	63
05/01	F	219.3	2	75.8	27.5	32.4	60.5
05/08	F	216.3	3	78.8	26.4	31.9	57
05/15	F	213.3	3	81.8	26.1	31.5	56
05/22	F	211	2.3	84.1	26.1	31.2	55
05/29	F	209.1	1.9	86	25.5	30.9	53.5
06/05	F	203.1	6	92	25.1	30	51
06/12	F	199.1	4	96	23.8	29.4	47.5
06/15	M	195	4.1	100.1	23.2	28.8	40
06/19	F	202.7					
06/26	F	199.9					
07/03	F	196.6					
07/10	F	197.7					
07/17	F	193.8					
07/24	F	192.2					
07/31	F	191.1					
08/05	W	189.9	5.1	105.2	20.8	28	39.5
09/04	F	188.6	1.3	106.5	20.9	27.8	39.5

Being 100% committed to this program and planning to succeed required establishing goals. Not just goals such as "I want to lose weight" or "I want to be healthy," but specific and outrageous goals. I hadn't weighed less than 200 pounds in over 20 years, so my first goal was just that — I'm going to weigh less than 200 pounds. Outrageous! Then I found out something else about Isagenix that I hadn't known before. They have a wall of fame and recognition program in place for everyone who releases 100 pounds or more from their body, regardless of time, if they used the Isagenix products to accomplish it. My next goal fell right into place — join the 100 Pound Club. Perfect! Even if I didn't win the IsaBody Challenge, I would have other recognition for my success that would help motivate me to maintain that success. That is an important point and you need to wrap your whole commitment into it. Success, no matter if it's measured in weight loss or some other aspect of your life, is not a destination that you arrive at and then you get to stop. *Success is a lifelong journey that requires commitment and a motivation to continue.* Make one of your goals something that will continue to motivate you for life. My goals were simple: Weigh less than 200 pounds. Join the 100 Pound Club. Win the IsaBody Challenge. Got it. Now let's get started.

Chapter 3
WHY ISAGENIX

Doctors get bombarded with emails, fliers, sales calls, and more about health information that will "change your life." Let's face it, over 80% of Americans are overweight in this unhealthy world and it's an enormous (no pun intended) global sales market. In addition to what comes through our offices, we have to watch the same television ads as everyone else that showcase their "results not typical" success stories. Most of us in the health and wellness industry become immune to the sales pitch and we've raised indifference to a whole new level. I was no exception. Even though my sponsor in Isagenix has a PhD in nutrition and is respected greatly by me and many others, I told him 'no' many times. I had seen too many programs and had tried too many systems to think that this one was any different. I was so indifferent that I didn't even do any research on the products offered by Isagenix and compare those products to everything else being promoted out there. What a colossal mistake on the part of any physician. Do your research. All doctors should clearly see after diligent research that everyone on the planet would benefit from the high quality of nutritional products offered through Isagenix. I'm embarrassed to say that I was arrogant about my own knowledge of nutrition and health simply due to the fact that one, I was a doctor and two, I teach a Human Anatomy & Physiology class for a local community college. I knew all there was to know — right? No. I was an obese know-it-all. In the end it wasn't even the nutrition that got me to use Isagenix products — it was about the competition of the IsaBody Challenge. I would ask questions later.

Once I started the Challenge, I started asking a lot of questions and I'm sure you can see why after you look at the following statistics. In the first 7 days I lost 12 pounds. *Interesting.* After 30 days, I had lost 32 pounds. *Hey, that's new.* After 80 days, 60 pounds had disappeared and I was feeling fantastic. *What's in this stuff?* My blood pressure dropped, my body fat percentage dropped, inches melted away, my stamina was boosted, and my skin glowed. *Holy cow!* In 24 weeks I had released a staggering 100 pounds and 98 inches and my body was still changing. *Are you kidding me!*

Take a look.

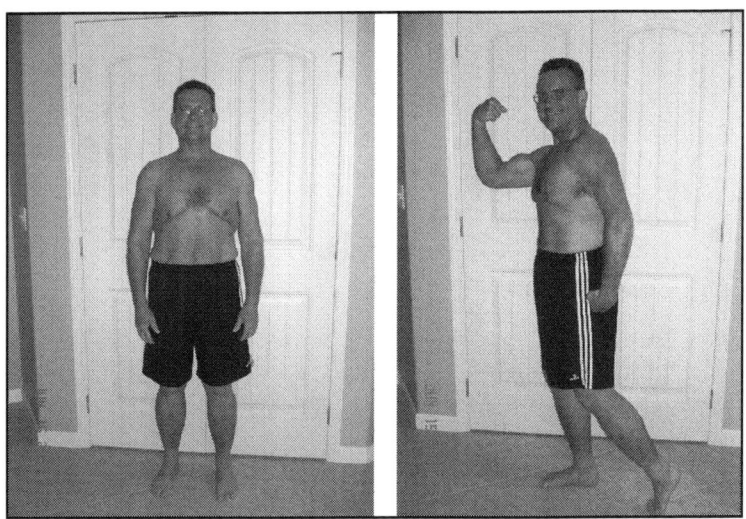

As a doctor using Isagenix products as a part of my Isa-Body Challenge, an entire library of questions opened that I soon found out had already been answered. If you take the time to research the pedigree of health and science professionals that directly contribute to the Isagenix program and products, you'll understand how absolutely foolish and arrogant I felt. Here is a list of websites where you can research this company and the professionals involved.

You'll be glad (and humbled) that you did.

IsagenixHealth.net - Our health and science newsletter is your hands-on, front-line resource for the latest news and product developments direct from our science team.

IsaHealthCoach.com - Provides coaching and training to make you as successful as you can be.

IsaProduct.com - Your quick link for access to the incredible line of Isagenix products.

IsaFYI.com - All of the latest and greatest information about products, incredible deals, breaking news, tips to build your business, and much more are now in one place online.

IsaDiary.com - Get the most out of Nutritional Cleansing with free advice.

IsaMovie.com - The most popular videos demonstrate how Isagenix transforms lives.

My results should not be considered typical. A 2008 university study showed a statistically significant weight loss of seven pounds during the first nine days of the Cleansing and Fat Burning System. As with any health or fitness program, a sensible eating plan and regular exercise are required in order to achieve long-term weight loss. I became active, made smart choices, and most important—I stuck to the program.

Chapter 4
WORKING THE SYSTEM

There are several systems available through Isagenix that promote healthy weight loss. The system in Isagenix that was recommended to me and that became the cornerstone of my success was the 30 Day Cleansing and Fat Burning System. This system uses a combination of meal replacement shakes perfectly balanced for the human body to release fat and gain lean muscle. I've never seen another meal replacement shake of this quality—ever. A cleansing nutrition vitally important for fat loss and health restoration is included. High antioxidant and active adaptogen combinations along with healthy snacks and other nutritional components designed for your success round out the system. It's the complete package, even if weight loss is your only goal. Since my goals eventually changed to include health maintenance and longevity, I have since included Isagenix Ageless Essentials in my program, as well. Here's a look at the way I used the 30 Day System for success.

30 DAY SYSTEM

Dr. Ken's Steps to Success

Shake Days

Note – A shake day and a pre-cleanse day are essentially the same thing. Your *minimum* water intake each day should be 64 fluid ounces. No excuses! Avoid carbonated beverages. To assist with calorie burning and weight loss, drink ice-cold water before meals. You will burn calories to heat the cold water to body temperature. To aid in digestion, room temperature water should be consumed after meals.

Special Note – When snacks are listed here, it's important to understand that the Isagenix Snacks and the IsaDelights have been formulated specifically for your success, especially on Cleanse Days. While I mention fruit as a snack option, it's important to understand that it was never my first option and I always tried to have organic, local fruit choices.

Breakfast

1 IsaLean Shake (I like them with 8oz water, 4oz crushed ice, and then blended)
1 Natural Accelerator

2 Hours Later (snack time at about 2 hours is crucial to keep the blood sugar stable)

> 2 Isagenix Snacks
>
> or 3–4 raw almonds
>
> or 1 IsaDelight (sold separately)
>
> or 1 medium apple (grapes, orange, banana, etc. okay, but not too much)

Lunch (90% of the time I chose lunch as my meal to keep me from eating too much at night without exercising.)

> Reasonable and healthy meal of 400–600 calories
>
> 1 Natural Accelerator

2 Hours Later

> Snack time as listed above.
>
> 1oz of Ionix Supreme (favorite time of day for me for energy boost and nutrition)

Dinner

> 1 IsaLean Shake

2 Hours Later

> Light snack such as Isagenix Snacks or almonds. It's best to stay away from fruit this late because of the sugar content without the exercise to burn it off before bed.

Bed Time

> 2 IsaFlush (These are important! They are not a laxative, but they help with regularity. They are mostly magnesium; a mineral incredibly beneficial to your heart and other organs. Don't skip these!) Check out the following study for regularity.

What promotes good bowel regularity? The CDC states, "It's recommended that you get 14 grams of dietary fiber for every 1,000 calories that you consume each day. If you need 2,000 calories each day, you should try to include 28 grams of dietary fiber."

Cleanse Days

> **Note –** This is a day set aside each week to detoxify the fat cells and other body tissues. It is an extremely important part of the 30 Day System when used for weight loss and other health issues. Follow it closely and make certain that you're drinking your minimum of 64oz of water. More is better, especially on a cleanse day.

Bowel regularity is of prime importance when an individual is cleansing. In the book, *Gut Solutions* by Brenda Watson, ND and Dr. Leonard Smith, MD, they state, "… *most holistic practitioners would consider the normal range of bowel movements to be one to three per day. The thinking here is that three movements would be ideal because we generally eat three meals daily.*"

Breakfast

4oz Cleanse for Life juice (try to drink at least 8oz of water after each cleanse drink to help with toxin removal)

1 Natural Accelerator

Snack (1½ hours after each cleanse worked best for me)

2 Isagenix Snacks

or 3–4 raw almonds

or 1 IsaDelight or 1 Isagenix SlimCake (both sold separately)

or 1 medium apple (grapes, orange, banana, etc. are okay, but not too much. 1 cup of raspberries, for example, is only 50 calories. Do your research.)

Late Morning

4oz Cleanse for Life juice

Snack

Same as above

Early Afternoon

4oz Cleanse for Life juice

1oz Ionix Supreme (still my favorite time of day)

1 Natural Accelerator

Snack

Same as above

Evening

4oz Cleanse for Life juice

Note – If you must, it's okay to eat a light and healthy salad. Make sure you keep it fresh and low calorie with lots of colors. A vinegar or lemon juice dressing keeps it low in calories and healthy.

Bed Time

2 IsaFlush

Special Note – It is documented in current text books (like the one I use to teach my Human Anatomy class) and journals that the correct amount of water intake for an active individual is 1 ounce of water for every 2 pounds of body weight. There are many opinions out there on this subject. This is the one I favor. Drink your water!

Dr. Ted recommended that I drink 2 glasses of cold water before each meal and each time I consumed the Isagenix Snacks. See facts below:

Water also plays a major role in appetite control. Here are the facts, Brenda Davy, associate professor in the Department of Human Nutrition, Foods and Exercise in the College of Agriculture and Life Sciences at Virginia Tech, who is senior author on the study, says, "We found in earlier studies that middle-aged and older people who drank 2 cups of water right before eating a meal ate between 75 and 90 fewer calories during that meal. In this recent study, we found that over the course of 12 weeks, dieters who drank water before meals, 3 times per day, lost about 5 pounds more than dieters who did not increase their water intake."

My purpose in this book is to draw your attention to the success you can envision in the IsaBody Challenge for yourself or for those you care about and to the Isagenix products—not to repeat what other health and wellness giants have already done before me. If you want more product information and research, I highly recommend a recently published book, *5 Minutes To Wellness* by Dr. Eric Kaplan.

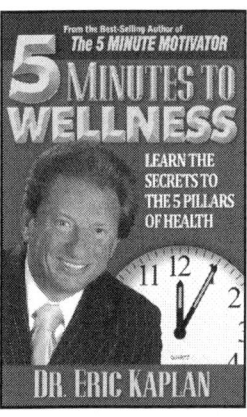

In it he writes, "...I began to research the company. I learned that Isagenix is more than a weight loss company, they offer an entire cleansing system, a toxin removal program, and a stress reduction system as well. ...The research provided here will show you how these products can help you restore your body's health by removing toxins, strengthening your tissues, and increasing your immune system while allowing your body to get its strength and stamina back."

It's a great book and I highly recommend you read it if only for the research and statistics alone.

Another great compilation of product information that I highly recommend is the brochure offered through Sound Concepts titled, *9 Secrets To Successful Cleansing And Weight Reduction*.

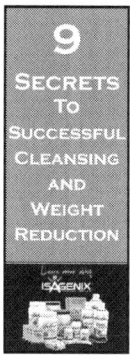

These articles weren't available to me during the 2009 IsaBody Challenge, but they are worth their weight in gold as are so many offered through both Sound Concepts and Isagenix. The research has already been done and it gives you the opportunity to stand on the shoulders of giants.

Chapter 5
COACHABILITY

I can't stress enough how important it is to listen to those who have been there before you and accomplished the goals they set out to achieve. We all think at some point that we don't need help, that we can do it ourselves. I'm sure I'm not alone in realizing that there is a reason that I had been overweight for over 20 years. I always thought I could do it myself, but that was a lie I told myself.

Accomplishing the goals I set for my-self was going to require some help this time—a whole lot of help—something I wasn't used to. Above all, I needed to be coachable. There are profession-als out there who have dedicated their lives to coaching others. Find one. For me it was the person who got me started in Isagenix. Since I first par-ticipated in the IsaBody Challenge they have implemented the IsaBody Challenge Mentor Program hosted by the fabulous Kjersti Cote.

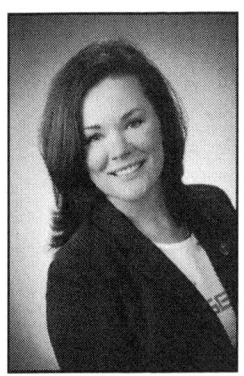

Kjersti Cote

They have a call you can listen to every Thursday at 6:30 p.m. PST where you get excellent coaching tips from numerous experts in all aspects of your journey. I rec-ommend accessing this call or its podcast recording at IsagenixPodcast.com whether you're in the Challenge or not. The information you learn from the various experts is invaluable. The number is 1-641-715-3842, Code 4000#. You can also check out the conference call schedule for other topics of interest depending on your goals. The pre-senters are amazing and all calls and recordings are de-signed to help you succeed.

I was a guest speaker on one of these coaching calls as a past Grand Prize Winner and was reminded of the importance of coachability when I heard what Mark Macey, 2007 IsaBody Challenge Grand Prize Winner, had to say about what he considered to be one of the most important keys to his success. He made the decision to be coachable and accountable to someone else.

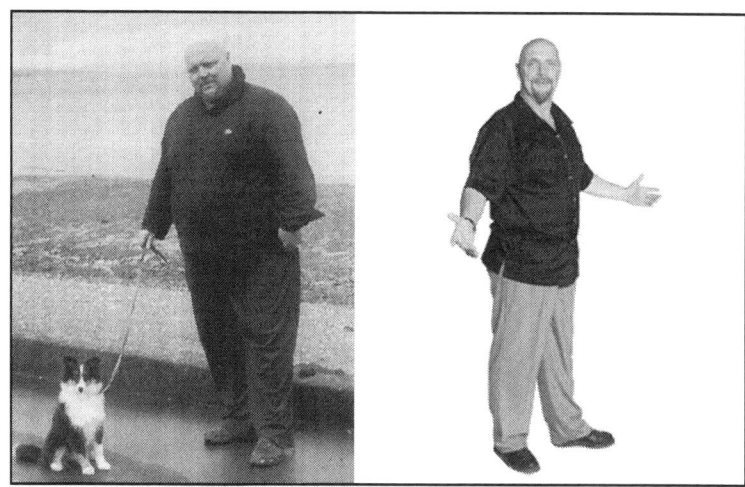

Mark Macey

Chapter 6
PLAN OF ACTION

The human body is in constant motion even at rest. It sounds funny to hear it put that way, but it is profoundly true. *Health is gained and maintained by action.* From the nutritionally dependent biochemical reactions and biological processes of each of our 70 trillion cells to the contraction and relaxing of our cardiac muscles 100,000 times a day, and everything in between, action is necessary for our survival. There is not one second of inactivity in our bodies, even when we sleep. There are, however, systems in our bodies that require muscular activity and purposeful movements for optimum health. Look at the lymphatic system, for example. The lymphatic system, a major player when it comes to our immunity, even lacks its own pumping organ as it relies largely on our actions and muscle contractions to propel its fluids. We were designed to move.

When we allow our lives to become sedentary, we cheat our bodies out of the way health should be. We must have a plan of action. For me, at 295 pounds, that was easier said than done. Even though I had my past athletic triumphs, action at this weight was going to be painful. To regain cardiovascular strength and endurance as 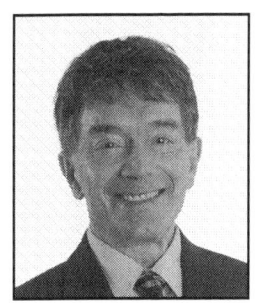 *Dr. Michael Colgan* well as calorie-burning lean muscle, some things needed to change. If you still don't fully understand the role that lean muscle plays in health and weight loss, I highly recommend the materials presented by world-renowned research scientist, Dr. Michael Colgan.

One of my favorite topics of his is his discussion regarding the importance of retaining lean muscle mass while losing weight, and why muscle just might hold the secret to successful and healthy weight loss for anyone. You can see here an example of the chart I used to document my movement on a daily basis.

My original plan was simple—move! A Duke University study found that "while 30 minutes of daily walking is enough to prevent weight gain in most relatively sedentary people, exercise beyond 30 minutes results in weight and fat loss. Burning an additional 300 calories a day with three miles of brisk walking (45 minutes should do it) could help you lose 30 pounds in a year without even changing how much you're eating." I set out to walk at a brisk pace for 30 to 45 minutes every day until I could do more strenuous activity. I really have my mother-in-law, Cherilyn, to thank for keeping me going and helping me follow through on my promise to move. She committed to walking with me every day and became my number one account-ability partner. When you know that someone is counting on you to be there, it makes it that much harder to quit. Find yourself an accountability partner for exercis-ing so you follow through on your promises to yourself. For me it was my mother-in-law and my fit-ness-conscious neighbors, Coach Ray and Dawna. For you, it may

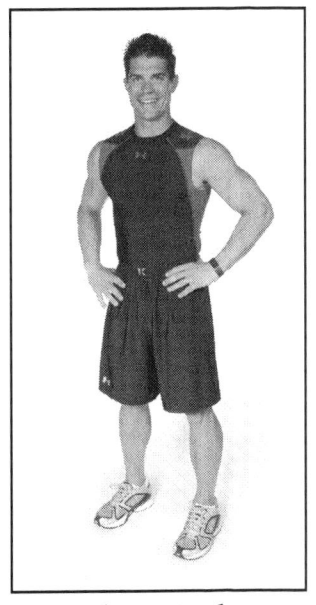

Shane Freels

be a personal trainer at a local gym or even group training like you can find at Camp Gladiator under the direction of Shane Freels.

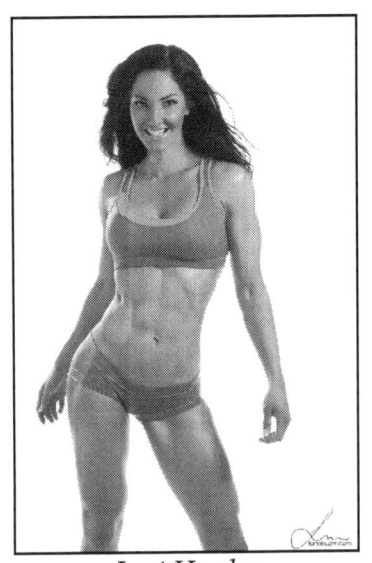

Lori Harder

If you set your goals high, you need to find someone to be ac-countable to that will bring out the best in you. I'm reminded of listening to the goals of 2010 IsaBody Challenge Grand Prize Winner Holly DeMott when she dreamed of posing in a bikini contest. Not only did she know that she needed to "get moving" as she put it, she went out and found a fit-ness trainer that could show her the way: Ms. Bikini Uni-verse, Lori Harder.

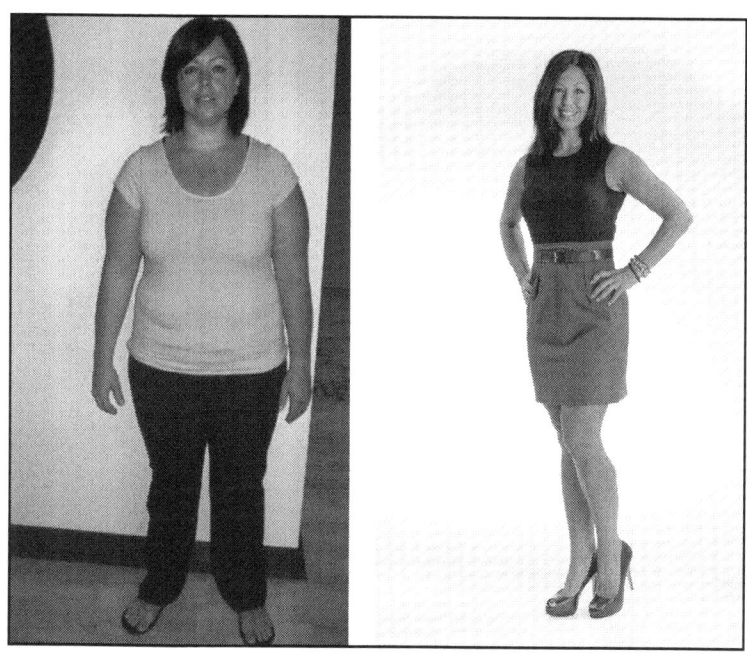

Holly DeMott

Chapter 7
NEVER GIVE UP

I mentioned earlier that I had to make a conscious decision every single day to succeed and for good reason. Quitting is easy. Quitting goes hand in hand with every excuse out there, and the more often you quit, the easier it gets — with only one exception: addictions. When you become addicted to something, quitting becomes seemingly impossible. Being addicted to food is no different than being addicted to other harmful items. Personally, I think food addictions are the worst and I'll tell you why I feel that way.

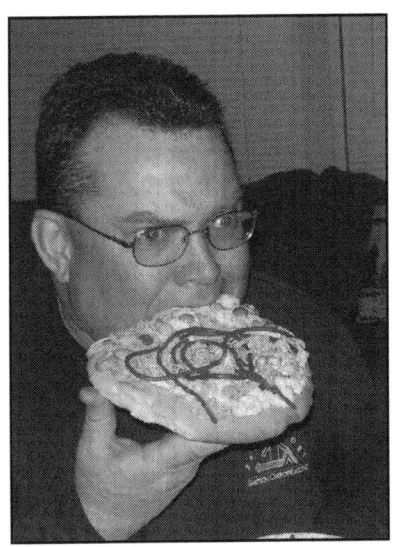

I'm going to pick on smokers for just a second, but only because smoking is number one in preventable causes of death each year because of its use and the effects of secondhand smoke. Being overweight or obese is currently in the second spot for causes of preventable deaths each year and is quickly gaining ground. According to the CDC (Centers for Disease Control and Prevention), approximately 20% of adults 18 years of age and older are smokers. Unlike food, however, smoking isn't necessary for our survival. Everyone has to eat to survive. We need calories and nutrition every day. You can't just quit eating to kick the habit of food addiction like you can so many others. We have to co-exist with food and change our relationship with food to make any reasonable change in our lives. This is a difficult task with fast food, processed food, and large portions so readily available. It's no wonder that over 80% of Americans are overweight, and one-third of all adults and one-sixth of all children are obese. I'm a doctor and I should've had a greater understanding of this, yet I've been both an obese child and an obese adult. Check out this excerpt taken from the book, *The UltraMind Solution*, written by Dr. Mark Hyman, MD. It helped me to regain control of what I was putting inside my body each day.

"The single biggest environmental influence you can control is what you eat. Remember, food is not just calories; it is information. It tells our genes what to do."

Our lives have become more sedentary, so we burn fewer calories. Also, we're eating more calories than we burn. Simple math shows that if you consume just 500 calories more each day than you burn, you're going to gain one pound of fat per week. That's 52 pounds gained in a year just because of a 500 calorie per day difference. We have to gain control of what we burn and what we consume. If we don't commit to controlling our caloric intake with balanced nutrition for optimum health and also exercising to gain and maintain lean muscle mass and cardiovascular strength, we're going to lose the battle. We have to make the necessary changes required to win our own personal battles and then — *never give up.*

I remember well the story of my new friend and the 2011 IsaBody Challenge Grand Prize Winner, Jill Birth, as she discussed her challenges with food addiction. She had tried to gain control over and over again to the point of having 24 sets of "before" photos and no "after" photos. She finally gained the upper hand in her battle, implemented Isagenix and the IsaBody Challenge to fuel her motivation, changed her relationship with food, and never gave up.

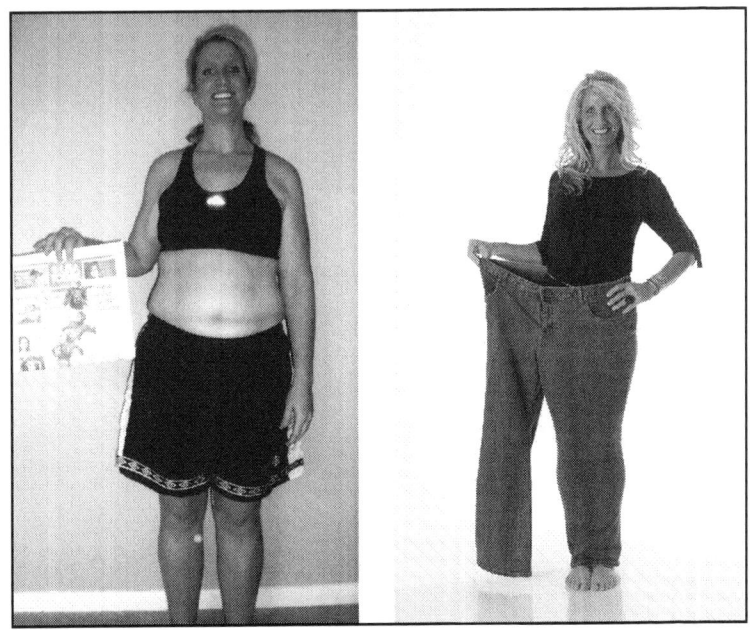

Jill Birth

Chapter 8
TESTIMONIALS

One of the things I absolutely love about the Isagenix products and the IsaBody Challenge is that the results *are* typical for those who make the commitment to change. Well over 250 individuals using the Isagenix products have joined the 100 Pound Club and many have joined the 200 Pound club and beyond with the number of members increasing regularly. Results become typical when they become easily duplicable, and Isagenix has certainly shown why they lead the world in the things that they do. If you want to be the best—align yourself with the best. I'm going to include some of my favorite testimonies. I want you to grasp the magnitude of success the IsaBody Challenge has created under the leadership of Rick Despain, Vice President of Field Development and all-around great guy.

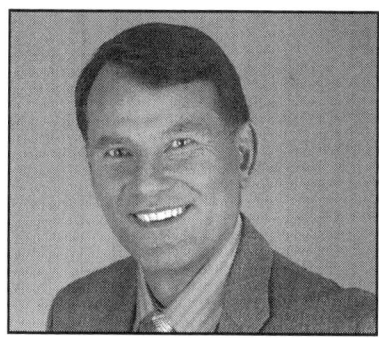

Rick Despain

If you need more evidence than the few testimonials I'm going to show you here, please go to the website, IsaBodyChallenge.com and select "Success". You can go through the years and amazing stories yourself and look at the difference the IsaBody Challenge has made in the lives of ordinary people.

Family Friendly

After Shelley Batson won 1st place in her category during the 2008 IsaBody Challenge, it inspired her husband, Bill and son, Keller to enter and subsequently win the 2009 Team category.

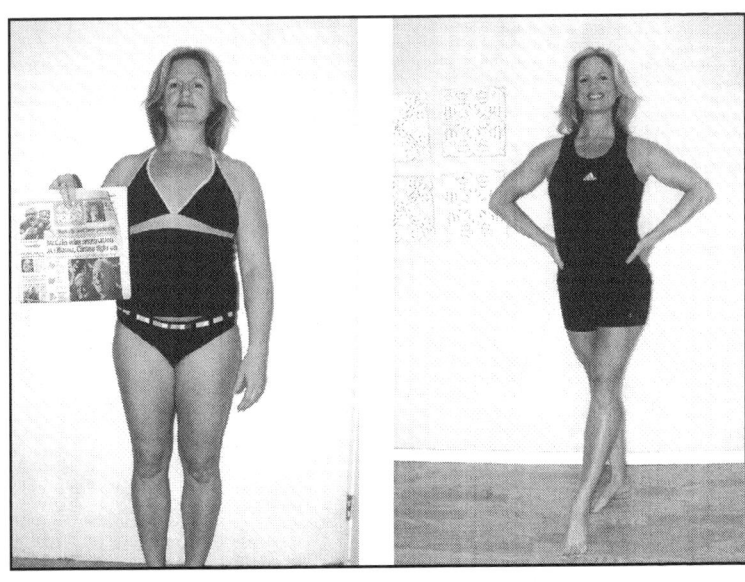

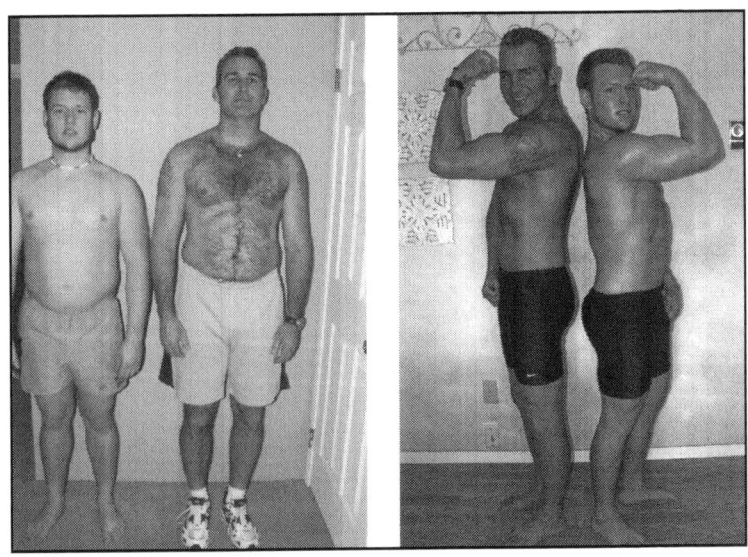

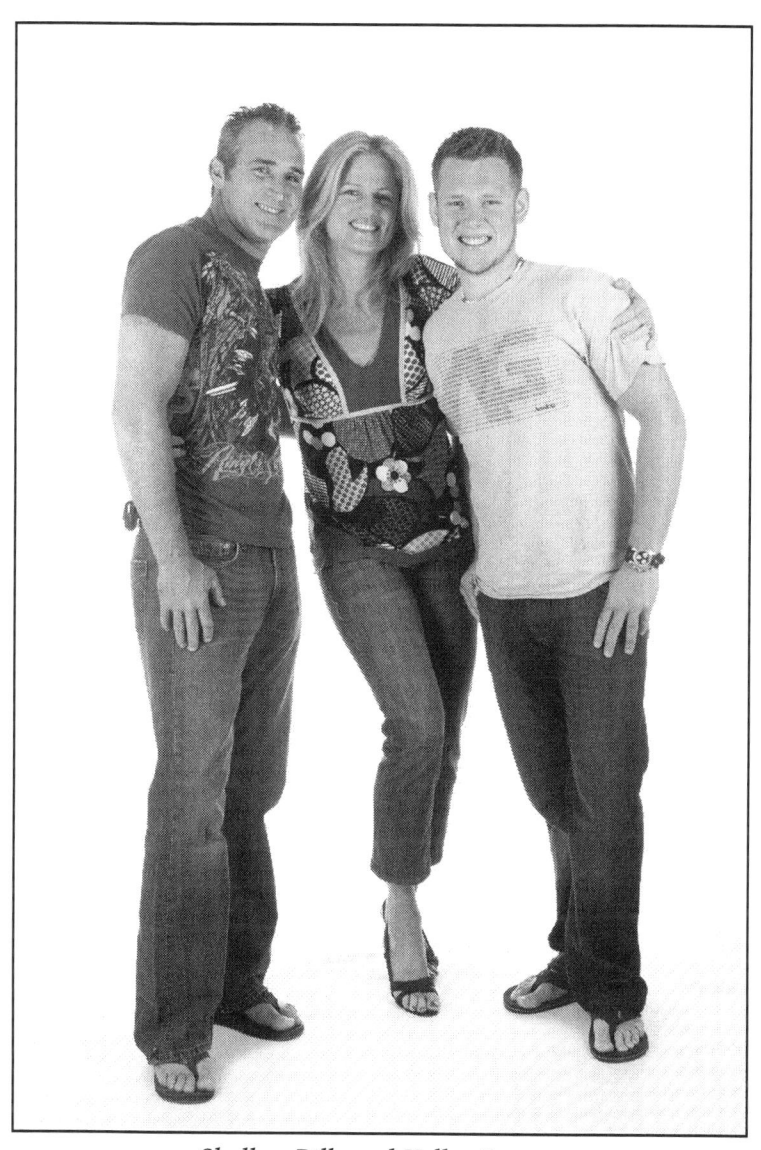

Shelley, Bill, and Keller Batson

Over 50? No Problem!

Take a look at Mark Douglas, Jean Faber, and Rick Kinmon. Mark reduced his weight by 50% and joined the 200 Pound Club even after struggling through a plateau on his way to two different IsaBody Challenge placings — 1st in 2009 and 3rd in 2011.

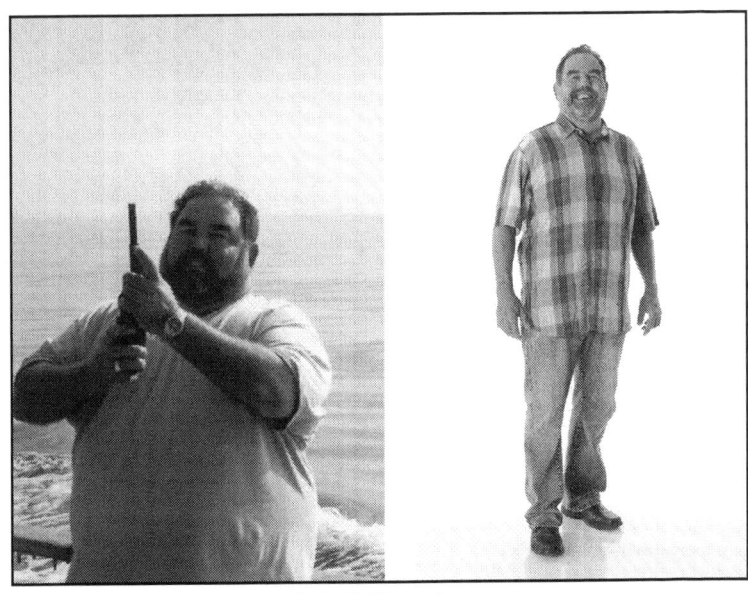

Mark Douglas

Jean has also released over 200 pounds and completely changed her relationship with food, going on to win 1st place in her category for 2010.

Rick battled joint pain from old injuries, but at the age of 59 he used the IsaBody Challenge and included in his routine the Isagenix product, Ageless Joint Support to change his physique and his circumstances. He placed 1st in the 50 and over category for 2011.

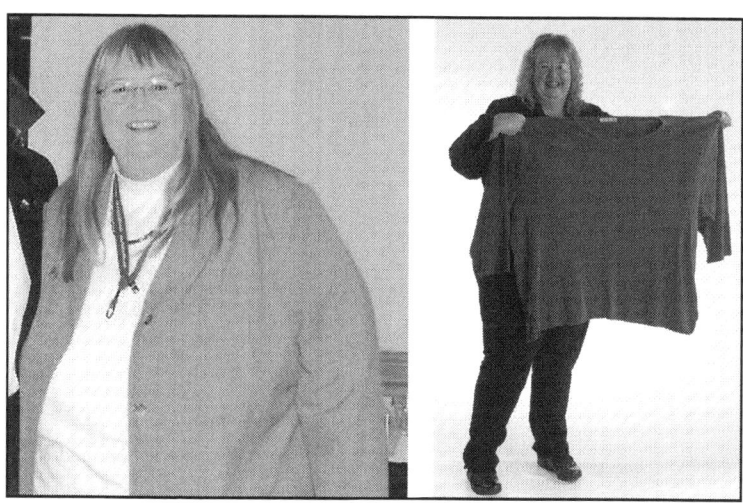

Jean Faber

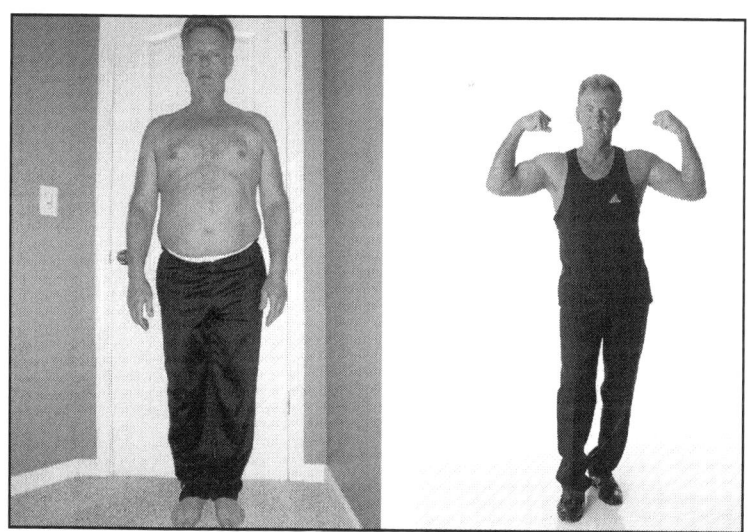

Rick Kinmon

Emotional and Physical Challenges

Whether shutting out the world or finally deciding against surgical procedures for weight loss, I'm very proud of contestants like Marina Bakker-Ayers, Oralia Alaniz, and Ryan Rhoades.

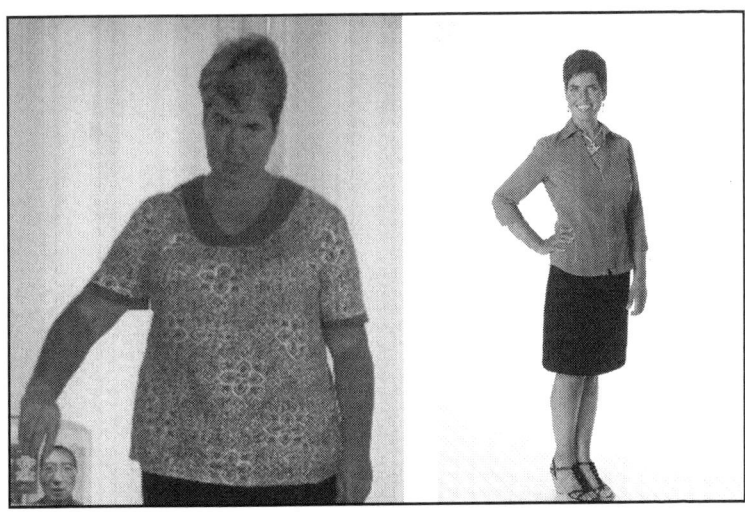

Marina Bakker-Ayers

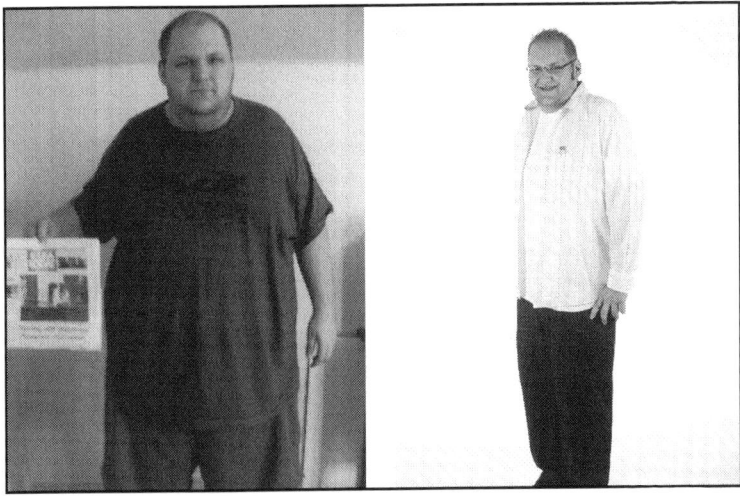

Ryan Rhoades

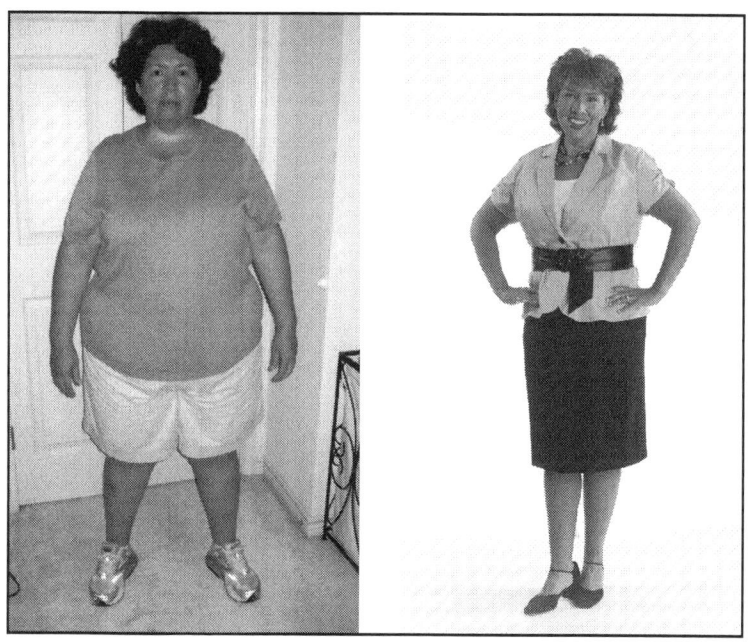

Oralia Alaniz

Young Guns and Fitness Fanatics

Check out Bruce and Theresa Coates, Kyle Symchysn and his mom, Pam Moore, and also Lisa Wolny. The muscular transformations of these bodies using this program are incredible. The IsaBody Challenge is not just about weight loss. It's about health, nutrition, and physical excellence!

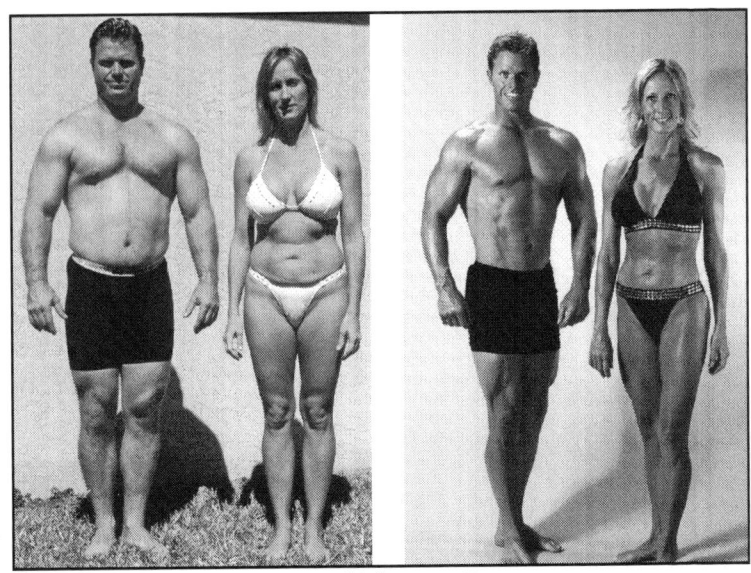

Bruce and Theresa Coates

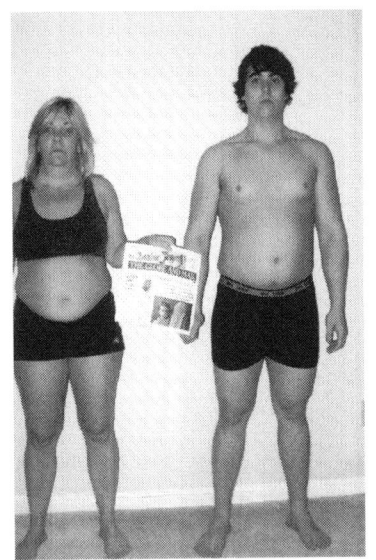 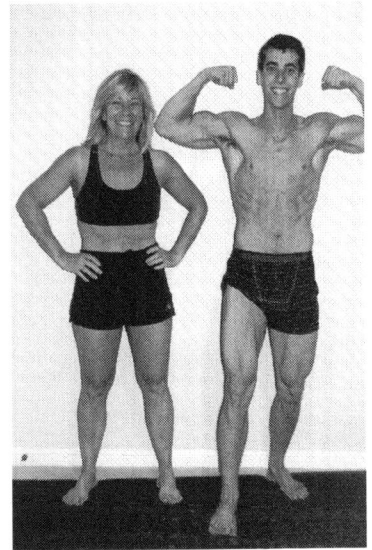

Kyle Symchysn and Pam Moore

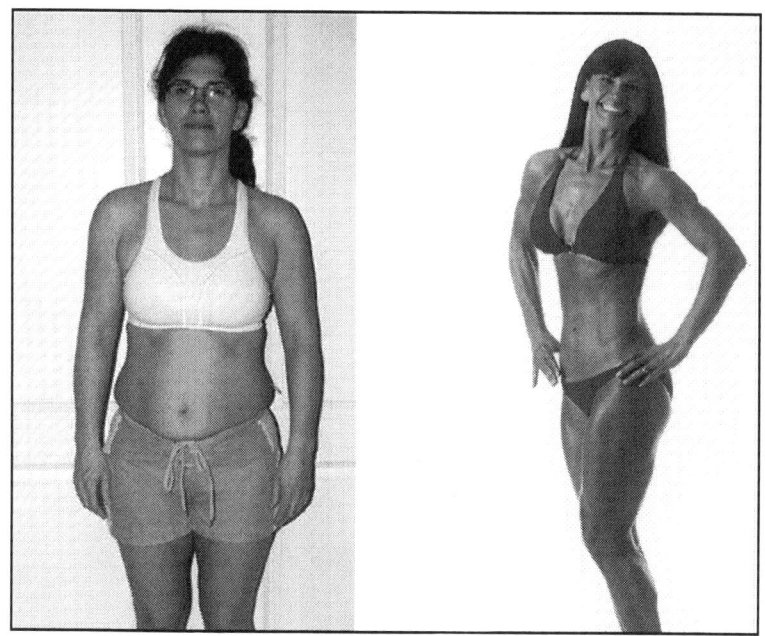

Lisa Wolny

Local Success

The IsaBody Challenge should be shared with friends and loved ones. I've always believed that something successful and life-changing should be shared. We all know someone who desperately needs change and every person on the planet needs excellent nutrition. Here are a few of my favorite local success stories out of the many that I have seen since beginning Isagenix. In fact, in 2011 I helped coach the release of over 2,000 pounds just from people in my community using the IsaBody Challenge and Isagenix. I threw a party celebrating their successes and many of those were able to attend.

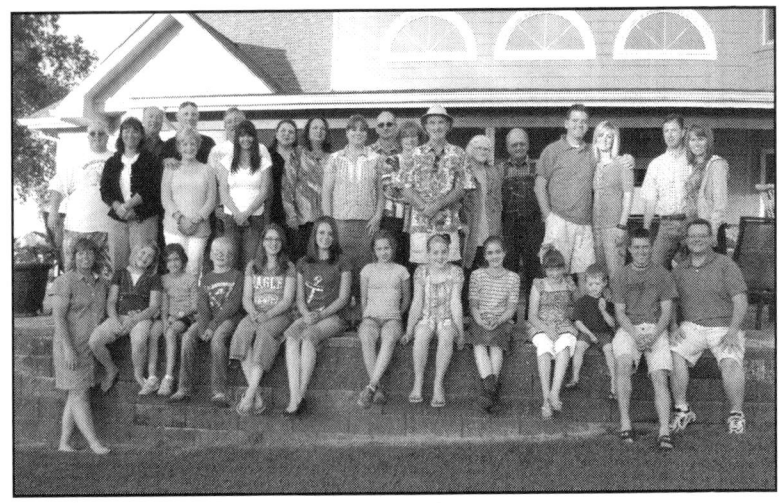

That's over 1 ton of fat gone! All four of the following lo-cal heroes had entries in the IsaBody Challenge as part of their motivation to change.

My friend and our high school principal, Ralph Brown weighed 270 pounds as early as the 7th grade, but found success and joined the 100 Pound Club because of the 2010 IsaBody Challenge and Isagenix.

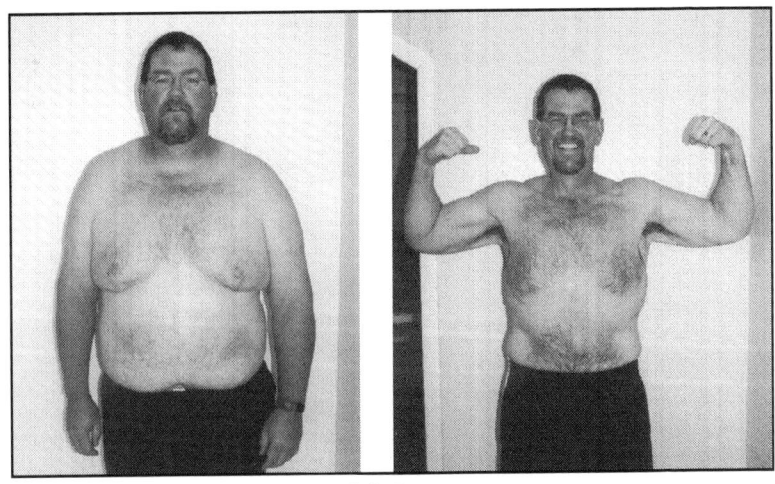

Ralph Brown

Mother of three and my lovely wife, Mindy decided to make a change during the 2011 IsaBody Challenge.

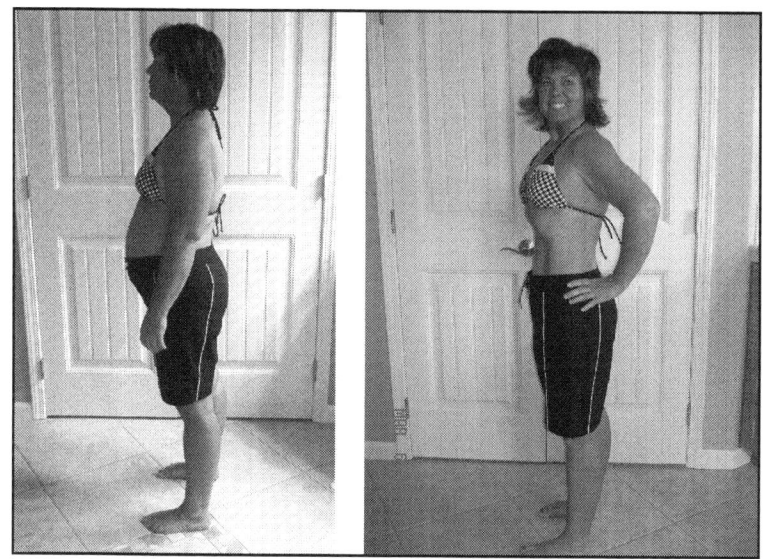

Mindy Simpson

My good friend and Vietnam War Veteran, Max Wells used the IsaBody Challenge as his platform for better health after being told by his doctor that he needed to drop 40 pounds and get his weight to 150 pounds to take better care of his heart.

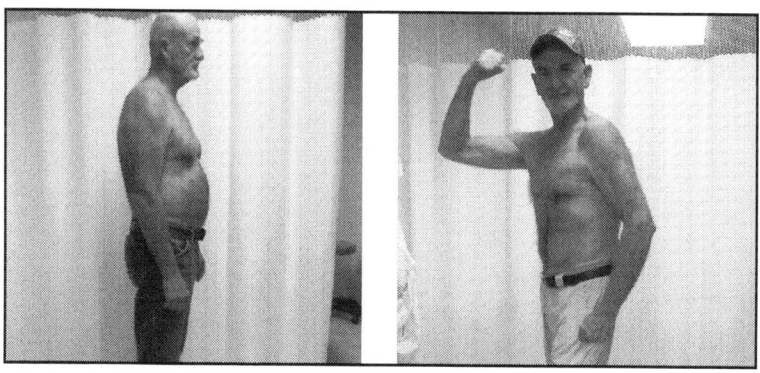

Max Wells

Local business woman, Rosie Knapp, described her life as barely existing before embarking on the 2011 IsaBody Challenge. After releasing 60 pounds and 61 inches, she now says she can't wait to get out of bed in the morning.

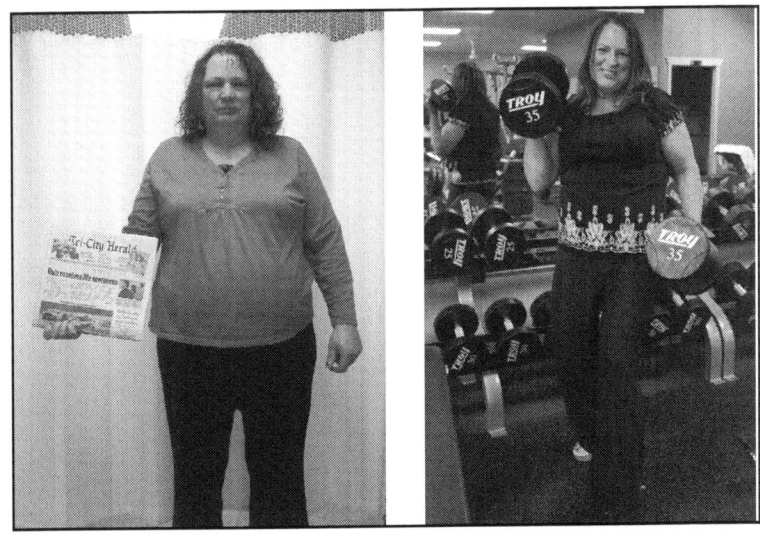

Rosie Knapp

Chapter 9
FROM PASSION TO PROFIT

Isagenix does not just help people succeed in life with body transformations alone. I would be neglectful in my desire to help others if I didn't mention that Isagenix has a program that also helps you find profit from your passion. There is a complete and unmatched financial reward structure by Isagenix that also recognizes individuals for their achievements — just by sharing the products and programs offered. Just by showing my friends, family and patients how to purchase their products at wholesale value and teaching them how to do the same with their friends, I now use my earnings from Isagenix to purchase 100% of the products used by me and my family with some "fun" money left over.

A winner in 2009 and 2011, Mark Douglas used his success in the IsaBody Challenge to catapult his financial success by teaching others to follow his example.

2011 IsaBody Challenge Grand Prize Winner, Jill Birth and 2011 2nd place age group winner, Lisa Wolny have taken it a step further in reaching out to others from all aspects of health and wellness and have escalated their financial gains as a result.

2010 Grand Prize Winner, Holly DeMott has traded in her corporate life for full-time financial rewards promoting Isagenix and has risen to a whole new level by building an entire network of fitness professionals as well.

In just their first 10 years, Isagenix has continued advancing in the nutrition and weight loss industry and has been featured in magazines, including making the cover of the

Fall 2011 Prosper magazine. In just 10 years, 62 associates have become millionaires using Isagenix and its compensation structure as their catalyst.

Whether your goals for transformation are physical, financial, or both, I have personally found that the opportunities for success are limitless with this company. I've only highlighted the successes of just a few that started their journey, me included, with the IsaBody Challenge. Please visit IsagenixBusiness.com for more information on how you can achieve financial success with Isagenix.

Chapter 10
CHOOSE HEALTH

The cold, hard reality of life is that it will throw you a curve ball when you're expecting a slider. Circumstances change that might make it more difficult to stay focused on your health and nutrition and old comforts and bad habits try to sneak their way back into your lifestyle. If we're not extremely careful with our choice of direction, we wake up one morning wondering why our clothes are too tight and our energy is low. It happens to the best of us when we lose control of our circumstances, even for a moment. My biggest stumble came in 2011 because of an accident I had when exercising. While on a bicycle ride with friends, I crashed into the pavement at 20 miles per hour (according to my GPS tracking device). My helmet was broken in three places, my bicycle was broken in at least that many, and I was a little broken myself.

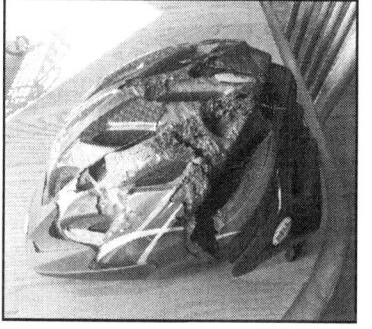

With a cracked rib, a cracked elbow, and several open wounds distributed evenly around my body just for balance, exercise was going to have to take a back seat for a while. I continued to make the Isagenix products a part of my everyday routine, but I wasn't exercising because of the scabs and the pain. When you consume more calories than you burn, you're going to gain weight. Remember? When you stop exercising you lose lean muscle mass and gain weight. Remember? I was guilty of both of those mistakes just because of a change in my circumstances. As soon as my injuries healed and I stopped feeling sorry for myself, I had to rekindle the desire to be where I was before the crash and get busy doing the right things again. I learned a very important lesson that we all need to face at some point in our lives. *Don't let circumstances stand in the way of your success!*

Let's revisit what I feel are the most important points I've made that could keep us healthy and successful through life's journeys.

1. **Enroll in Isagenix.** Enter the IsaBody Challenge, or encourage a friend or family member to do so, and help them stay on track. Whether or not you think you or they can win makes no difference. Everyone who makes this event a part of their journey is a winner. (And let's not forget the cash, the prizes, the free products, or the cruise!)

2. **Throw away your excuses**. Look where they've gotten you thus far. It's time for a change and you're the only one who can make the decision to do it.

3. **Make a conscious decision every day to succeed.** The right mindset means everything in life.

4. **Success is a lifelong journey**, not a destination. Don't let a change in your circumstances get in the way of your success.

5. **Find a goal that motivates you** to continue along the right path for the rest of your life.

6. **Do your research**. You need to be on board 100% — no doubts, no questions. These products are world leaders and you need to be aware of that and commit to them wholly.

7. **Be coachable**. If you haven't been able to make a change by yourself before, don't think your results will be any different if you try this time. Learn to trust others and be accountable. If you don't have a local accountability partner, look online. A University of Vermont study found that online weight loss buddies help you keep the weight off. The researchers followed volunteers for 18 months. Those assigned to an Internet-based weight maintenance program sustained their weight loss better than those who met face-to-face in a support group.

8. **Get moving**. We were designed to move. Schedule your exercise and make it a priority.

9. **Never give up** on your goals and dreams. Quitting should never be an option. Quitters never win and winners never quit.

10. **Choose health** by choosing the Isagenix products and the IsaBody Challenge. It's time to be addicted to having good health, and this company, what it stands for and promotes, is your golden ticket. Seize it!

Thank you for taking the time to read this book.

Go to **IsaHealthCoach.com** if you have any more questions or wish to contact someone regarding what you've read here. My prayer is that this work will help your decision to change your life and those around you that so desperately need change.

Now go and unlock the champion inside you!

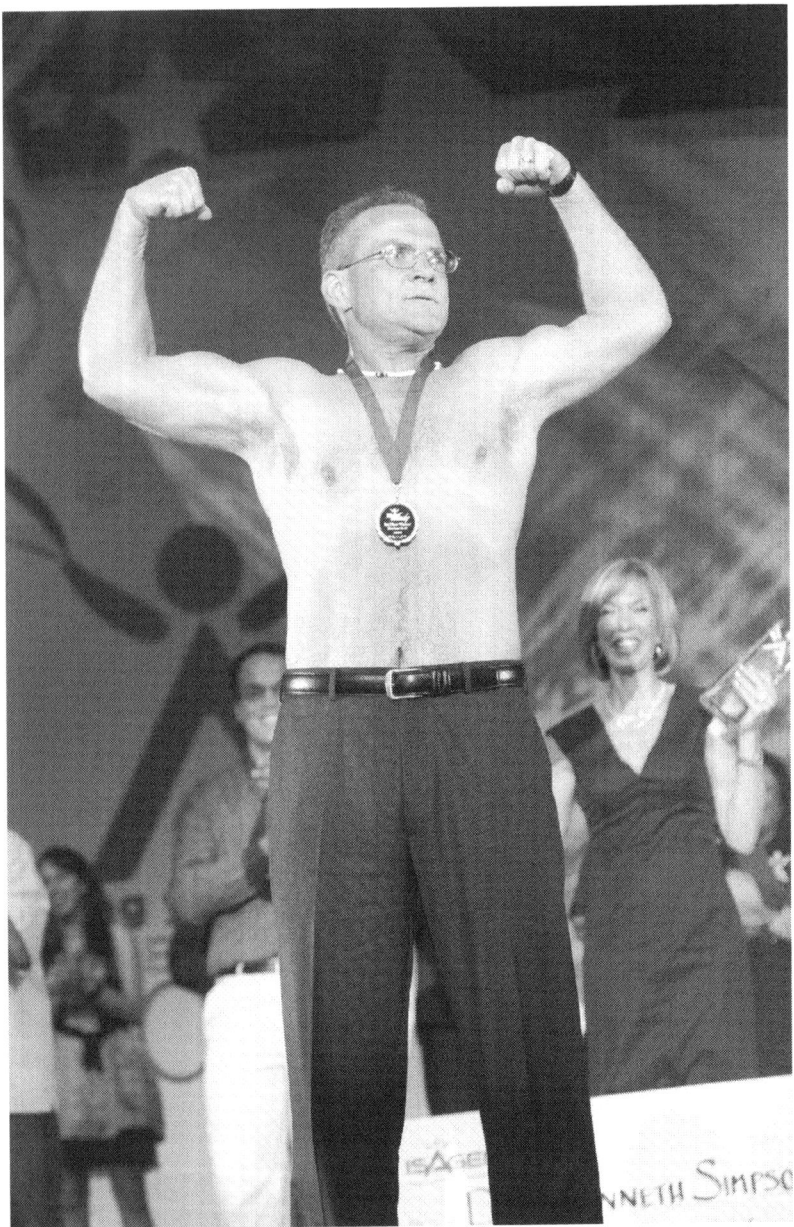

Dr. Ken Simpson, 2009 IsaBody Challenge Grand Prize Winner

Made in the USA
Lexington, KY
23 April 2014